5 Main Causes of Cancer

Things that stimulates malignant growth in the body

Susan Linda

Table Of Contents

Presentation

Meaning of Disease and how destructive it could be

Disease is a sickness where a portion of the body's cells develop wildly and spread to different pieces of the body. Disease can begin anyplace in the human body, which is composed of trillions of cells. Ordinarily, human cells develop and increase (through an interaction called cell division) to shape new cells as the body needs them. At the point when cells become old separates, and strange or harmed cells develop and increase when they shouldn't. These cells might frame growths, which are chunks of tissue. Growths can be harmful or not malignant (harmless).
Destructive growths spread into, or attack, close to tissues and can make a trip to far off places in the body to frame new cancers (a cycle called metastasis). Destructive growths may likewise be called dangerous cancers. Numerous malignant growths structure strong cancers, however tumours of the blood, like leukemias, by and large don't.

Harmless growths don't spread into, or attack, close to tissues. At the point when taken out, harmless cancers for the most part don't come back, while malignant growths some of the time do. Harmless growths can at times be very enormous, notwithstanding. Some can cause serious side effects or be perilous, like harmless growths in the cerebrum.

Malignant growth is the second most normal reason for death in the U.S. In any case, less individuals are passing on from malignant growth now than a long time back. Early location and creative therapies are restoring malignant growth and assisting individuals with disease live longer. Simultaneously, clinical specialists are recognizing autonomous gamble factors connected to creating malignant growth to assist with keeping individuals from creating disease

According to the American Cancer Society, 1 in 2 men and people assigned male at birth (AMAB) and 1 in 3 women and people assigned female at birth (AFAB) will develop cancer. As of 2019, more than 16.9 million people in the U.S. were living with cancer. The most common cancers in the United States are:

Breast cancer: Breast cancer is the most common type of cancer. It mostly affects women and people AFAB. But about 1% of all breast cancer cases affect men and people AMAB.
Lung cancer: Lung cancer is the second most common cancer. There are two types of lung cancer: non-small cell cancer and small cell lung cancer.
Prostate cancer: This cancer affects 1 in 9 men and people AMAB.
Colorectal cancer: Colon cancer and rectal cancer affect different parts of your digestive system.

Blood cancers: Leukaemia and lymphoma are the most
common

Disease begins when a quality or a few qualities change and
make dangerous cells. These cells make disease groups, or
cancers. Malignant cells might split away from cancers,
utilising your lymphatic framework or circulatory system to
make a trip to different regions of your body. (Medical services
suppliers call this metastasis. For instance, a cancer in your
bosom might spread to your lungs, making it difficult for you to
relax. In certain kinds of blood disease, unusual cells in your
bone marrow cause strange platelets that duplicate wildly. In
the end, the unusual cells swarm out typical platelets.

Chapter 1

Your age

Malignant growth can require a very long time to create. That is the reason a great many people determined to have disease are 65 or more seasoned. While it's more considered normal in more established grown-ups, malignant growth isn't solely a grown-up sickness — disease can be analysed at whatever stage in life.

The more established we get, the more probable we are to foster malignant growth. Many individuals are astonished by this.

Anecdotes about kids or youngsters with disease will generally stand out as truly newsworthy, as they are much of the time the cases which are the most surprising. Be that as it may, getting malignant growth very early on is intriguing.

1 out of 2 individuals will get disease in the course of their life - one of the fundamental explanations behind this being that individuals are living longer. A big part of all diseases are in individuals beyond 70 years old.
However, ageing doesn't mean you will get malignant growth.

Age is the most elevated risk factor for fostering a greater part of malignant growths, with a couple of exemptions.

According to the National Cancer Institute (NCI), the median patient age at the time of a cancer diagnosis is 66. The majority of cancer patients — 60% of them — are 65 or older. In fact, one-quarter of new cancer cases are diagnosed in people between the ages of 65 and 74. And the most common cancers occur more often in older patients. The median age for breast cancer is 61; for colorectal cancer, it is 68 and for lung cancer, it is 70.

Maturing increases disease gambles in our bodies in more ways than one. The more established we are, the higher the extent we get of cells with changes. Also, these cells make populaces of high gamble for selecting malignant growth starting cells.

As years pass, we amass our openness to hurtful things that can add to malignant growth risk: the UV radiation, destructive synthetic substances, remembering those for tobacco smoke and infections.

A subsequent explanation maturing expands our malignant growth risk is that as we age, we experience a downfall of our invulnerable capabilities, which, while functioning admirably, offer us steady reconnaissance and destruction of cells that are suspected to become harmful.

A third explanation likewise has a place with resistant framework failing: in the old, their safe frameworks are continually on a bogus self-alert (called persistent foundational sterile irritation) and this makes conditions that animate duplication of cells from high-risk populaces, consequently inciting their change into malignant growth cells.

First and generally significant, we want to comprehend and track down ways of getting maturing to stretch out an individual's capacity to stay solid. Current science is hugely moving toward improvement of maturing treatments. Fully expecting these arising arrangements, which are supposed to cordially change what is happening to better, we can in any case help ourselves by pursuing sound life routines to dial back maturing and consequently decrease the gamble of malignant growth. These incorporate following a sound eating regimen, consuming cell reinforcements and treating persistent irritations.

Other than preventive measures, the best anticancer safeguard is schooling and readiness: realising that malignant growth risk increments as we age, we want to follow suggested disease early-location strategies and know about advances we might have to take on the off chance that we truly do get disease and have to pick a therapy routine.

My colleague Grace Dy, MD, Professor of Oncology in Thoracic Medicine, says that while living longer exposes us to more wear and tear on our bodies, "age alone does not determine what treatments to give in general.

Chapter 2

Your Habit

Certain way of life decisions are known to build your gamble of malignant growth. Smoking, drinking more than one beverage daily for ladies and up to two beverages per day for men, exorbitant openness to the sun or regular rankling burns from the sun, being fat, and having hazardous sex can add to disease.
You can address these habits to bring down your gamble of malignant growth — however a few habits are simpler to change than others.

Smoking can cause disease and afterward block your body from battling it;

Harms in tobacco smoke can debilitate the body's resistant framework, making it harder to kill malignant growth cells. At the point when this occurs, disease cells continue developing without being halted.
Harms in tobacco smoke can harm or change a cell's DNA. DNA is the cell's "guidance manual" that controls a cell's typical development and capability. At the point when DNA is harmed, a cell can start outgrowing control and make a disease grow.
Specialists have known for quite a long time that smoking causes most cellular breakdowns in the lungs. Today's

actually obvious, when almost 9 out of 10 cellular breakdowns in the lungs pass through by smoking cigarettes or handed-down cigarette smoke exposure. Truth be told, individuals who smoke have a more serious gamble for cellular breakdown in the lungs today, despite the fact that they smoke less cigarettes. One explanation might be changes in how cigarettes are made and what synthetic compounds they contain

Smoking can cause disease anyplace in your body, including the:

Blood (intense myeloid leukaemia)
Bladder
Cervix
Colon and rectum
Throat
Kidney and renal pelvis
Larynx
Liver
Lungs, windpipe, and bronchus
Mouth and throat
Pancreas
Stomach
Men with prostate disease who smoke might be bound to pass on from prostate malignant growth than nonsmokers.

The main thing you can do to forestall smoking-related malignant growth isn't to smoke cigarettes, or to stop on the off chance that you do. Staying away from handed-down cigarette smoke is additionally significant.

Stopping smoking brings down the gamble for 12 kinds of
malignant growth: tumours of the lung, larynx, oral pit and
pharynx, throat, pancreas, bladder, stomach, colon and
rectum, liver, cervix, kidney, and intense myeloid leukaemia
(AML).

Within 5-10 years of stopping, your possibility of getting
malignant growth of the mouth, throat, or voice box drops
significantly.
In something like 10 years of stopping, your possibility of
getting malignant growth of the bladder, throat, or kidney
diminishes.
Inside 10-15 years after you quit smoking, your gamble of
cellular breakdown in the lungs drops significantly.
In something like 20 years after you quit smoking, your
gamble of getting malignant growth of the mouth, throat, voice
box, or pancreas drops too close to that of somebody who
doesn't smoke. Additionally, the gamble of cervical malignant
growth comes around about half.

Smoking causes at least 15 different types of cancer and is
the biggest cause of lung cancer in the UK as researched by
CANCER RESEARCH UK

The sex act has numerous medical advantages from
diminishing pressure and strain, to supporting your
insusceptible framework. It might try and influence your
gamble of fostering specific diseases.

In any case, likewise with most matters of wellbeing, how sex
and malignant growth risk are connected is convoluted and
reliant upon a few elements. Your age, orientation, and how
frequently you practise safe sex will all impact your potential
malignant growth risk.

Until this point, the main clear writing connecting sex and malignant growth is that unsettling the human papillomavirus (HPV). There are north of 200 types of HPV, yet some are more malignant growth causing than others. Fortunately we currently have an immunisation against the most widely recognized malignant growth causing kinds of the infection.

Most generally, HPV is connected to cervical malignant growth. In any case, all kinds of people can expand their gamble of creating disease through sexual exercises that pass on the infection.

Chapter 3

Family ancestry

Disease is normal - many individuals have somebody in their family who as of now has or has had malignant growth. It is entirely expected for more than one individual from a family to have disease.

Disease can happen in families:

just by some coincidence, which is most frequently the situation
since relatives have the equivalent natural and way of life risk factors, for instance an excess of sun or smoking, or
since there is an acquired flawed quality which builds the gamble of malignant growth, which is phenomenal.
Just a little level of specific diseases (up to 5%) are because of a defective quality acquired from either the dad or mother. This is the very thing that we call a familial or family disease. This can likewise be alluded to as an acquired inclination to disease. The broken quality builds the gamble of malignant growth, yet and, after its all said and done, it doesn't mean each relative will foster the disease.

 Check out at the family ancestry on both your dad's and your mom's side of the family. The enlightens that diseases the

family might be because of an acquired defective quality
include:

Number of blood relatives* who have had disease
The more blood relatives* who have had malignant growth
(specifically bosom, ovarian or potentially entrail disease), the
more probable the malignant growth is because of an
acquired broken quality.

Ages at which tumors in the family created
The more youthful individuals were the point at which they
created malignant growth (contrasted with what is generally
anticipated in the overall local area), the more probable it is to
be because of acquired factors.

Example of disease in the family
The sort of disease and who it influences in the family are
significant. In certain families there are various blood
relatives* who foster a similar sort of disease, like bosom or
entrail malignant growth. In different families there are a few
diseases that might run in the family (for example bosom,
ovarian or inside malignant growth and disease of the uterus).
This happens on the grounds that a few broken qualities can
cause more than one kind of disease.

The more hints that are available, the more probable it is that
there is an acquired defective quality in the family causing a
higher than common possibility of malignant growth. Be that
as it may, it isn't clear. It is critical to realize that certain
individuals who acquire a defective quality which causes an
expanded gamble of malignant growth never proceed to foster
disease.

*A close family member is somebody related by blood (for example grandma, father, sister), not marriage.
Most diseases are brought about by quality blames that occur during our lifetime

Certain individuals have an expanded gamble of specific sorts of disease since they have acquired a broken quality

Your PCP can allude you to a hereditary centre on the off chance that you have serious areas of strength for a background marked by disease

A few defective qualities that increment the gamble of disease can be given from parent to kid. These are acquired disease quality issues. They happen when there is a shortcoming in the qualities in an egg or sperm cell at the hour of origination. These flaws in the underlying sperm or egg cell are replicated into each and every cell in the body. The broken qualities can then pass from one age to another. They are called germline transformations.

We acquire qualities from both our folks. In the event that a parent has a quality shortcoming, every youngster has a 1 out of 2 possibility (half) of acquiring it. Thus, a few kids will have the defective quality and an expanded gamble of creating malignant growth and a few youngsters will not.

Being brought into the world with acquired defective qualities doesn't imply that an individual will get disease. Yet, they have a higher gamble of creating specific sorts of disease than others. They are likewise bound to foster disease at a more youthful age. Specialists call this having a hereditary inclination to malignant growth. For a malignant growth to grow, further quality changes (transformations) need to occur. This generally occurs over numerous years.

In the event that you have a family background of bosom, ovarian, uterine, or colorectal malignant growth, you might have a higher gamble for fostering these tumours.

Let your primary care physician know if :

A relative was determined before age 50 to have uterine, bosom, or colorectal malignant growth.
At least two family members on a similar side of the family were determined to have uterine, bosom, or colorectal disease.
A female relative was determined to have ovarian malignant growth.
A male relative was determined to have bosom malignant growth.
You have an Eastern European or Ashkenazi Jewish family line.
Enlightening your primary care physician concerning your family wellbeing history is the initial step to see whether you might have a higher malignant growth risk. It could assist you and your primary care physician with concluding what tests you want to evaluate for disease, when to begin, and how frequently to be tried. Knowing your family wellbeing history likewise assists you and your primary care physician with choosing if hereditary guiding or testing might be ideal for you.

Chapter 4

Obesity

Overweight and stoutness can cause changes in the body including enduring aggravation and higher than ordinary degrees of insulin, insulin-like development variable, and sex chemicals. These progressions might prompt malignant growth. The gamble of malignant growth increases with the more overabundant weight an individual increases and the more extended an individual is overweight.

Corpulence has been connected to a few normal diseases including bosom, colorectal, esophageal, kidney, gallbladder, uterine, pancreatic, and liver malignant growth. Stoutness likewise builds the gamble of kicking the bucket from malignant growth and may impact the treatment decisions. Around 4-8% of all diseases are credited to weight. The basic system of heftiness causing malignant growth is complicated and is deficiently perceived. Way of life changes that incorporate eating routine, exercise, and conduct treatment are the pillar of intercessions. Drug treatment and weight decrease a medical procedure bring about a more quick weight reduction and might be utilised for a subgroup of disease survivors with stoutness.

There are three essential organic components that have been proposed as a gamble of the improvement of threat in stout people . The first of these components is connected with the idea of fat tissue going about as an "organ", with the ability to deliver substance arbiters and compounds. In particular, this system depicts expanded amalgamation of estradiol from androgens because of the presence of aromatase tracked down in fringe fat tissue. The overproduction of oestrogen by fat tissue has been connected to an expanded gamble of creating bosom, endometrial, ovarian, and different diseases.

The subsequent component is the outcome of hyperinsulinemia because of expanded BMI, which animates the typical development capability of insulin as well as drawing out the span of the activity of insulin-like development factor-1 (IGF-1). Insulin and IGF-1 blood levels are oftentimes higher in corpulent individuals. Insulin obstruction, one more settled disease risk factor, causes high measures of insulin, or hyperinsulinemia, which happens before the beginning of type 2 diabetes. The improvement of colon, renal, prostate, and endometrial malignant growth might be helped by high insulin and IGF-1 levels.

The third piece of the component connects with the proinflammatory climate developed by the modified emission of numerous adipokines (polypeptide chemicals) by fat tissue, explicitly expanded degrees of leptin, which is a strong provocative, proliferative, and hostile to apoptotic agent.Adiponectin, which is another adipokine that has antiproliferative properties, is low in large people with a solid weight. Abundance of fat tissue prompts adipocyte hypertrophy and cell passing bringing about the persistent, subclinical irritation of fat tissue. A few pre-clinical examinations support that constant irritation in fat tissue triggers cancer-causing agents and the movement of malignant growth. People with overabundant body weight have modified degrees of provocative cytokines including

IL-6, TNFα, and C-responsive protein. The predominance of constant provocative sicknesses, including gallstones and non-alcoholic greasy liver illness, is higher in large grown-ups. These elements make oxidative pressure, which harms DNA and makes individuals bound to foster biliary plot, liver, and different malignancies. Weight may likewise build the gamble of malignant growth by lessening cancer invulnerability and modifying the mechanical qualities of the tissue that encompasses developing cancers . Adipokines, resistant cell adjustment and fundamental irritation, angiogenesis, metabolic changes, extracellular framework regulation, and extracellular vesicles, for example, exosomes have been embroiled in metastases

Many individuals generally tend to assume that weight gain and heftiness are brought about by an absence of self control.

That is not completely evident. Despite the fact that weight gain is generally a consequence of eating conduct and way of life, certain individuals are in a difficult spot with regards to controlling their dietary patterns.

Indeed, indulging is driven by different organic variables like hereditary qualities and chemicals. Certain individuals are essentially inclined toward putting on weight.

Obviously, individuals can defeat their hereditary drawbacks by changing their way of life and conduct. Way of life changes require self control, commitment and diligence.

By the way, claims that conduct is absolutely an element of determination is very oversimplified.

They don't consider the wide range of various variables that eventually figure out what individuals do and when they do it.

A few factors that are driving reasons for weight gain, heftiness and metabolic illness, a large number of which don't have anything to do with determination.

1. Hereditary qualities
Stoutness has serious areas of strength for a part. Offspring of guardians with corpulence are substantially more prone to have weight than offspring of lean guardians.

That doesn't imply that weight is totally foreordained. What you eat can significantly affect which qualities are communicated and which are not.

Non-industrialized social orders quickly foster corpulence when they begin eating a common Western eating regimen. Their qualities didn't change, yet the climate and the signs they shipped off their qualities did.

2. Designed Unhealthy Foods
Vigorously handled food sources are many times minimal more than refined fixings blended in with added substances.

These items are intended to be modest, keep going long on the rack and taste so staggeringly great that they are difficult to stand up to.

By making food sources as delicious as could really be expected, food producers are attempting to increment deals. Be that as it may, they likewise advance by indulging.

Most handled food sources today don't look like entire food varieties by any means. These are profoundly designed items, intended to get individuals snared.

3. Food Compulsion
Many sugar-improved, high-fat unhealthy foods animate the reward communities in your cerebrum.

As a matter of fact, these food sources are frequently contrasted with normally mishandled drugs like liquor, cocaine, nicotine and weed.

Low quality foods can cause enslavement in defenceless people. These individuals let completely go over their eating conduct, like individuals battling with liquor compulsion letting completely go over their drinking conduct.

Fixation is a complicated issue that can be undeniably challenging to survive. At the point when you become dependent on something, you lose your opportunity of decision and the natural chemistry in your mind begins giving orders for you.

Eating great and being more dynamic are the most effective ways to work on your wellbeing assuming that you are overweight or corpulent. Losing just 5% to 10% of your all out body weight can lessen your gamble of creating disease. It might appear to be a limited quantity, however research demonstrates the way that it can work on your wellbeing. Regardless of whether you find shedding pounds hard, eating a more adjusted diet and practising consistently assists bring down your disease with gambling.

Here are a few things you can do to assist you with pursuing better decisions:

Pursue little changes in your food decisions and work-out daily practice. Assuming that you battle with being more dynamic and eating less, individuals from your medical services group can help. An enrolled dietitian, practise subject matter expert, therapist, or specialist who spends significant time in weight reduction are experts who can assist you with making changes.

- Get support: It is vital to feel upheld while attempting to make life changes. Most health improvement plans incorporate meetings with a dietitian or weight reduction trained professional. They can assist you with rolling out better improvements and stick with them over the long run. Converse with your family about the progressions you need to make and request that they help. It is a lot simpler to make changes in the event that individuals you live with make them, as well.

- Prescription: Some medical services suppliers might suggest taking prescription in the event that eating routine, exercis don't work and your heftiness is causing other serious ailments.

Chapter 5

Environmental causes

A few synthetics in the climate are harmful substances that can deliver malignant growth in people and creatures. Most synthetic substances act by causing the commencement step in the malignant growth process (modifying the DNA), however they likewise can go about as advertisers.

Various synthetic substances are uncovered to be perilous at high fixation synthetic compounds to our wellbeing. These disease causing specialists are called cancer-causing agents. We have in excess of 100,000 synthetic components in our current circumstance in which 30,000 of them have been dissected. Out of 30,000 dissected ones, simply 275 of them ended up being cancer-causing. Individuals who have specific positions, for example, painting, development, pesticide and petrol labourers have an expanded gamble of disease. Many examinations have shown that openness to asbestos, benzene, benzidine, cadmium, nickel, arsenic, radon and vinyl chloride in the working environment can cause disease. The investigation of physiological irregularities during fetal advancement is called teratology which is brought about by natural substances called teratogens. Fundamentally, a teratogen goes after the foetal genome and can bring about different deformations. Four manifestational aggregates can happen, for example, contortion (congenital fissure), development hindrance (anencephaly), practical deformity (ventricular septal imperfection) and demise. Around 10% of all birth absconds are made by pre-birth openness teratogenic specialists which incorporate medication, maternal contaminations, natural and word related openings. Nonetheless, multifactorial cooperations of teratogens and human hereditary inconstancy can add to the singular degree of limit defenselessness. Arsenic is profoundly harmful to human tissues, bugs, microbes and organisms. Polluted groundwater with metallic arsenic has caused arsenic harming for a large number of individuals around the world. Arsenic has been related with heritable changes in quality articulation, for example, DNA hypermethylation of cancer silencer qualities, histone adjustments and RNA impedance. Arsenic trioxide has been endorsed by FDA in 2000 to be utilised for intense promyelocytic leukaemia (APL) and psoriasis . As of late, the arsenic has been utilised in pet sweep (a positron producer) for better imaging. Mutagen is a natural, physical or synthetic cancer-causing specialist that can change the hereditary structure of a cell. A few gathered hereditary transformations can change an ordinary cell to a dangerous one. A few changes are caused suddenly during cell fix, replication and recombination without the mutagenic effect. The mutagens and delivered free revolutionaries can be taken out from body tissues by powerful cell reinforcements, for example, nutrients A, C, E, polyphenols, Flavonoids and selenium components

The expression "climate" incorporates air, water, and soil, yet additionally substances and conditions in the work environment, schools, home, and different spots individuals live, work, and play.

The main dangers of creating disease come from way of life factors. Nonetheless, openings to specific human-made and normally happening synthetic compounds in the climate might add to a singular's gamble of creating malignant growth. Benzene, asbestos, vinyl chloride, radon, arsenic, and trichloroethylene are instances of poisonous substances that can build the gamble of disease when individuals are presented to them.

The Worldwide Organization for Exploration on Malignant Growth (IARC) has ordered these substances (and numerous others) as known human cancer-causing agents. A few different synthetics have been displayed to cause malignant growth in creatures, yet there isn't sufficient proof to show these synthetic substances cause disease in individuals. These synthetic compounds are arranged by IARC as could be expected or plausible (thought) human cancer-causing agents. The sort and measure of openness to destructive synthetic substances impacts the gamble of creating disease .